# The 8 Eating Rules

# The 8 Eating Rules
Lose Weight and Improve Your Health…One Habit at a Time

by Stavros Mastrogiannis

Live Your Way Thin Publications

## Dedication

This book is dedicated to the fight against obesity and to the millions of people who are trying to balance life, weight loss, and staying healthy. The purpose of this book is to provide these people with the ammunition they need to finally win their weight loss battle.

## Disclaimer

The author recommends talking to your doctor and getting a full physical before starting any exercise and/or diet program. The medical community has varying opinions on proper nutrition, improving health, and losing weight. This book contains the opinions of the author, and is for reference and informational purposes only. It is in no way intended as medical counseling or medical advice. The activities, physical or otherwise, described herein are for informational purposes only, and may be too strenuous or dangerous for some people. Please consult with your doctor before engaging in them. The author and the publisher cannot be held liable for any injury caused, or alleged to be caused, directly or indirectly, by the information contained in this book.

# Table of Contents

# Foreword

I had become skeptical about weight loss. With all the wild claims out there, can you blame me? Most of us have heard of programs that promise us that by simply using a particular, targeted exercise or by eating only certain foods, all our health issues will be solved. But, through failed attempts and simple reasoning, we have come to find there are no "magic pills" for weight loss. I had settled into a place in my life where I would discount any fitness program as being unsound and that weight loss and good health were things I was predisposed not to be able to obtain.

Because I felt defeated, it took me over a year after I had heard of the success of Stavros's program before I finally decided to meet with him. When I took a closer look, I saw that Stavros's program did not make any promises of magical cures. He explained that weight loss was a matter of slowly adjusting my behavior to relearn how to eat. He explained that it had to be a gradual process. I was impressed with the fact that his program was not a sales pitch. He did not try to trick me into joining a club or making purchases in a food program. He stated the facts, as he does in this book, and then it was up to me.

When I began the program, I weighed 268 pounds and had health problems that included high blood pressure, high cholesterol, and pre-diabetes. I had seen family members battle the severe outcomes of these conditions, therefore I felt a certain urgency about losing weight. At times I became impatient and wanted to move faster and lose weight more quickly, but Stavros would explain that week-to-week weigh-ins were not the main focus, but rather the goal was a lifetime of fitness.

Stavros's program was not overwhelming and didn't cause me to burn out. For the first couple of months, weight loss was steady and gradual. On occasion I lost focus and became distracted, but my weight remained steady. When I refocused on the rules of the program, the weight began to come off again.

There were also times I stumbled on a certain Eating Rule. These were short setbacks, however, and they did not derail the lessons I had already put into practice. If I slipped back into old ways for a day or for one meal, it was not the end of the program. Most of the time there was a lesson to be learned as to why I ate improperly.

The hints for recognizing cravings and dealing with them were a huge aid. If I was craving a particular food, I had to hold off only until the weekend and, most times, by the time the weekend came, the craving had long passed. If I was eating because of stress or any other emotional reason, I learned to identify this compulsion and deal with the stress in a different and much healthier manner.

With Stavros's help, I realized that weight loss occurred naturally, due to the combination of muscle gain from strength training, the slow burn of fat from cardio, and the replacement of foods that cause weight gain with foods that promote good nutrition and digestive health.

Over seven months, I lost over 40 pounds of fat, and gained muscle and flexibility. My blood pressure and cholesterol stabilized and my blood glucose level returned to normal. I gained much more energy and I didn't get heartburn or feel bloated every day, particularly after meals. I had more progress to make, and continued to incorporate these new behaviors and attitudes into my life.

Today I feel healthier, I know that I've achieved good, long-lasting results, and I know I will continue to see the benefits of healthful eating. Now that I've established these new eating and exercise behaviors, it would be difficult to change back to constantly eating for reasons other than for being hungry.

I wholeheartedly recommend this book and this program to anyone who is tired of yo-yo dieting and is serious about losing weight and keeping it off. Because of the success that I have found, I can say without hesitation that if you follow this program, you can achieve your long-term fitness goals, and you, too, will be successful.

*Grant Rogers*

# Introduction

I have been in the weight loss field for over 17 years. I have seen so many people go on a diet, lose weight, and then regain the weight. When I ask people about the diet they used to lose weight, many times they tell me the diet worked when they were on it, but they simply couldn't stay on it any longer. It seems that most of the available diet programs are interested in helping people lose weight fast, but not permanently. This is one reason why, despite the millions of diet books sold every year in the U.S., we are still losing the weight loss battle.

Before you start thinking this is just another diet book, I want you to know up front, it is not. There are two main differences between this book and all other diet books. The first difference is that I will not ask you to give up junk food and other "bad" foods you may enjoy eating. In this book I will teach you how to live with those foods and still lose the weight you want and improve your health.

The second difference is that you'll learn much more than merely what you should eat in order to lose weight and improve your health. You'll learn how to eat, and, most importantly, how to incorporate this advice into your life so it becomes habitual, because permanent weight loss only comes through making permanent changes in your habits.

My dietary advice is not based only on what I learned in school. As matter of fact, a lot of the things I learned about "proper" nutrition were wrong. To further my education, I looked at many cultures, including where I came from — Greece, where people live long and healthy lives. I looked at hundreds of nutritional studies and, more importantly, I looked at who did the studies, since studies can be manipulated. I also used common sense to determine what information made sense and what did not. For example, most nutritionists will tell you breakfast is the most important meal of the day. That advice never made sense to me and, as you will learn in this book, breakfast is *not* the most important meal. You'll learn why it isn't, and what is.

As I said before, weight loss and improved health are not just about knowing what eating habits you need to have in order to lose weight. You must know how to make those eating habits become *your* eating habits, without overwhelming yourself. This book you will teach you, through 14 Simple Steps, how to develop the right eating habits and make the 8 Eating Rules part of your life so you will lose *all* the weight you want and, more importantly, keep it off for the rest of your life.

*Stavros Mastrogiannis*

## Section 1: Weight Gain is a Blessing

You're probably thinking I have lost my mind, but once I explain why weight gain is a blessing, I'm sure you will agree with me. Many people believe that because they are thin, they don't have to worry about their diet — that only people who have a weight problem need to think about what they eat. These thin people should think again. Being thin does not mean junk food has no ill effects on you. All it means is that your body can burn, or not observe, the extra calories, so your weight does not increase. However, you still can develop heart disease, diabetes, or any other disease that overweight people develop.

The reason I consider gaining weight a blessing is the fact that, at the very least, people who gain weight when they eat poorly and/or don't exercise get a clear message in the mirror that tells them, *you are doing something wrong*, whereas a thin person often does not get that message until it's too late.

Due to the fact that thin people don't see any dramatic physical consequences in the mirror because of bad eating habits or lack of exercise, often a thin person will find it much harder to improve his or her diet and start an exercise program than someone who gains weight easily. A thin person doesn't have that extra motivation to look good in a bathing suit because he or she looks fine now, and can't see what bad habits are doing to their health on the inside.

So you see, if you are overweight and you gain weight easily, you should consider yourself lucky to have an obvious advance warning that's telling you to take action *now*.

# Section 2:
# Why We Can't Keep Weight Off
# After We Lose It

These days we can't turn on the TV or look at a magazine without seeing an ad for some weight loss product or service. One would think, with all those weight loss products and services on the market today, we would be the thinnest nation in the world, but we're not! Americans spend billions of dollars per year on weight loss products and services, and yet we are still losing the weight loss battle. There are many reasons why we have not been able to lose weight, or to be more precise, to lose weight and keep it off. Here I will talk about what I consider the number one reason for this.

I would like to start with a question. What is the one thing most weight loss products and services on the market today have in common? They promise fast results. The reason they promise fast results is because that's what people want to hear. They don't take into consideration the fact that fast results are almost impossible to maintain for the long term, but then again, the ads only promise that we will lose the weight fast, not that we'll be able to keep it off. Most weight loss products can deliver on their promise of fast results, but where they fail miserably is in delivering permanent results.

Let me explain the reason why they fail at helping people lose weight permanently. Here is an undisputed fact: In order to lose weight fast, you must make big changes in your life. There is no way around this fact. The problem with big changes is that they take us far outside our comfort zone. The farther away you get from your comfort zone, the more likely you will get overwhelmed and quit.

Humans are creatures of habit. The majority of the things we do every day require little or no active thought on our part. When we do the things we have always done, things we know we can do, we are inside our comfort zone. If we want to change our habits, or add a new habit, we need to take ourselves out of "automatic gear" and consciously practice the new habit, which requires more energy on our part. Whether that energy is mental or physical does not matter, because either way, when we're trying to implement a new habit in our everyday lives, that new action takes us outside our comfort zone, which makes us feel uncomfortable, and our bodies fight to get us back into the comfort zone. Of course, by repeating the new action, eventually the comfort zone expands to include that new action.

The question is, can you keep repeating the new action and tolerate the discomfort long enough for that new action to become a habit and get within your comfort zone? Also keep in mind that the more new habits we're trying to develop at once, the bigger the discomfort we will feel and the longer it will take for our comfort zone to expand to include the new habits, which means we have a greater chance of burning out. It's important to implement change one small step at a time.

Unfortunately, most weight loss programs and diets on the market today simply don't understand how habits are formed and how people's comfort zones work — or they just don't care, because all they want is to make a quick buck. They wrongly assume that once we start seeing results we'll be motivated to stick with their diet or weight loss program. Wrong! If results were enough to motivate us, then why can't most people keep the weight off after they lose it? Statistics show that the vast majority of people regain lost weight within four to five years.

The main reason we regain the weight is because most weight loss programs and diets ask us to make many big changes all at once. They fail to understand how to introduce and apply change into our lives without overwhelming us. They have no understanding of how to best eliminate or develop habits, and that is why most weight loss programs and diets fail. This book will not only tell you what actions to take for better health and permanent weight loss, it will also teach you how to develop those actions into everyday habits.

# Section 3: How to Lose Weight and Keep it Off

The best way to lose weight is through small, sustainable changes over time. All the actions required to lose the weight have to become automatic *habits* and part of your comfort zone — if you want to keep the weight off. Actually, the process of losing weight permanently is much easier than losing weight quickly, because you only need to make small changes at any one time. Each week your focus should be on the habit or habits you are trying to develop, not the weight. In Section 8, you'll learn how to introduce good eating and physical activity habits through 14 Simple Steps. As you're working through the steps, it's important to remember that your excess weight is only a symptom of a problem. The true problem is the habits that made you overweight in the first place.

By following the 14 Simple Steps, you'll lose weight more slowly, but you will only need to lose the weight once, whereas with most of the weight loss programs and diets on the market today, you'd end up having to lose the same weight over and over again every year. What's the point of losing weight fast, if you're going to gain it all back again? Wouldn't you rather take a few extra months, lose the weight the right way, and never worry about your weight again for the rest of your life?

## Section 4: Saying No to Junk Food Can Hurt Your Weight Loss Goals

First of all, let's talk about what I mean by "junk food." My definition of junk food is any food that is highly processed, high in refined carbs (white flour and/or sugar), has little or no nutritional value, and that is eaten for the sheer pleasure of it. Examples of junk foods include, but are not limited to, white bread, cake, ice cream, doughnuts, cookies, milkshakes, high-sugar salad dressings and dips, soda, candy, desserts, chips of any kind, most alcoholic drinks (more than one per sitting), etc. By the way, merely adding vitamins to a food does not take it off the list of junk foods.

The one thing most diets have in common is that they want you to eat certain foods and completely eliminate others, usually junk foods. However, these diets don't take into account the human psychology behind wanting something you can't have. Have you ever watched a child play with one toy while completely ignoring another toy lying nearby? As soon as another child picks up that toy, all of a sudden the first child wants it. It's human nature to want what we can't have, therefore trying to eliminate certain foods only draws attention to the foods we can no longer have. And let's face it; most "bad" foods taste good.

Most diets tell you to eliminate all junk food from your diet so you can lose weight fast. Most people do exactly that, and lose weight. However, since we often want what we can't have, it's only a matter of time before we give in to an inevitable craving.

When we do, we say to ourselves, "I cheated already. I feel guilty anyway, so I might as well have all the junk food I want today. Tomorrow I'll be extra good to make up for today."

That is how binge eating starts. The fear of not being able to have a certain food can cause us to binge on that food. Before we know it, we start breaking the diet more often, especially when the scale starts moving up. We eventually give up, and by that time, we may even have established a habit of binge eating.

So you see, by simply saying "no" to junk food, all we do is make ourselves want it even more. If it were that easy to give up junk food, the junk food companies would be out of business by now! But they're not, because it's not that easy to give up junk food. However, as you will learn in this book, you won't have to. The 8 Eating Rules include guidelines for the times and places when your favorite "bad" foods are allowed.

# Section 5: Control Yourself, Not Your Environment

Another big mistake we make when trying to lose weight is cleaning out our cupboards. We eliminate all the foods we're not supposed to eat by getting them out of the house. I even hear nutritionists recommending this approach, with the idea that their clients will not be tempted to cheat. This sounds like good advice on the surface, but it does not teach us one very important thing: self-control.

I lived in Greece for 12 years before moving to the U.S., at which point, over a long period and before I knew any better, I picked up many bad eating habits. I never had a weight problem, but when I got into the fitness field I realized that not gaining weight didn't necessarily mean that junk food had no ill effect on my body. That's when I tried to change the bad eating habits I had picked up over the years.

On my first attempt, I did what most people do. I eliminated from my house all my favorite junk foods and sodas and told myself I would never have them again. The problem I found with this method was, every time I encountered my favorite junk foods somewhere else, say, at a party, I would binge on them. After eating only one piece of food that was on the "forbidden" list, I'd tell myself, "Oh well, I broke my rule. Might as well enjoy all the junk food I can have now, and tomorrow I will be extra good with my diet to make up for today."

This would happen two or three times each week because, as you know, junk food is everywhere. In this way, I learned that trying to control my environment (in this case, by removing all the junk food from my house) does not work.

I started looking at people who were successful, not just in weight loss, but in business and in life, and what I found out was this: People who are successful in their endeavors don't eliminate all temptation from their lives. What they do is learn to make themselves to do the right thing, in spite of all the temptations around them.

Weight loss is no different. You must learn to control yourself, not your environment, because the fact is, you can't always control your environment.

You can eliminate all the tempting foods from your house, but can you do the same for your work environment? Most people that I've talked to say this is not possible, since co-workers frequently bring candy and other sweets to share at work.

So my question then became, how can I learn to control myself? It took a little time, but after a few more failed attempts, I came up with a method by which I was able to take complete control of my eating habits, and had absolutely no problem resisting food temptations of all kinds. I could go to a party where they had all my favorite sweets, have a great time, and not have even one sweet. Most importantly, I did not feel deprived. I kept all my favorite cookies in my house without feeling the urge to eat one. Here's how I did it.

It started with the realization that having *some* junk food will not kill us. After all, we ate junk food in Greece when I lived there and we were very healthy and thin. My school in Greece had about 350 kids and, out of all those kids, only three or four were overweight. I thought cancer was a rare disease because I didn't know anyone — or even know anyone who *knew* anyone — who had cancer. The average 80-year-old person was completely independent and fully functioning; I had never seen a walker and not even many canes. People lived long and healthy lives, and yet still ate some junk food.

But here is the difference: We did not eat it every day. We usually reserved it for special occasions. For instance, about once each week, when there was a good movie on TV, my mother gave us potato chips and Coke as a snack to eat during the movie. Although there was always soda at our celebrations and holiday parties, there was no soda during our regular lunch or dinners. There was no dessert after dinner — only when we went to a restaurant did we have dessert. At home, dessert was usually apples or oranges. Only on holidays did my mother make those delicious Greek desserts, like baklava and galaktoboureko.

Nowadays if you go to Greece, people have become very overweight, including the kids. What changed? Among other things, junk food has gone from being a treat eaten once in a while to something indulged in every day, many times instead of a regular meal.

The point I'm trying to make is that we don't need to eliminate all the junk food from our lives to be thin and healthy. All we need to do is treat junk foods as they were meant to be treated — as a treat. In other words, we need to make junk food special, like it used to be. Once I realized that, I was able to come up with a plan to help myself put junk food in its proper place in our diet, as a treat. Here's how I made junk food special again.

I started with soda. I was a very heavy soda drinker, and knew that if I simply tried to eliminate soda from my diet, it wouldn't work — cravings would sabotage my effort. Instead, I made a rule that I could not have any soda Monday through Friday, but I could have all the soda I wanted on weekends, starting at 5 p.m. on Friday. This made my weekend more special. I told my family — and I have a big family — that I would be required to give $20 to anyone who saw me drinking soda, including diet soda, during the week before 5 p.m. on Friday.

The first week was hard, but because I could have all the soda I wanted on the weekend, I found it much easier to resist temptation during the week. Whenever I had a craving for soda, I said to myself, "I should wait to have soda this weekend so I can enjoy it, without feeling guilty about it afterwards."

That first weekend, I drank plenty of soda to make up for not having it all week. I must say, I enjoyed my soda much more because I did not feel guilty about drinking it. On Monday, again I stopped drinking soda until 5 p.m. on Friday. This time it was much easier to resist drinking soda.

Whenever I felt a craving, I dismissed it as soon as it came up. I said to myself, "It's a weekday, and on weekdays I don't drink soda." I didn't dwell on the fact that I could not have the soda I craved. I just moved on, and thought about something else, or engaged in an activity that left no room for thoughts about the food I craved. I found that by dismissing the craving right away, the craving lost its power over me.

That weekend I drank soda again, but not as much as I'd had the previous week. Once I became comfortable with the knowledge of being able to have all the soda I wanted every weekend, I did not have the urge to drink soda during the week. When Monday came around, not having soda was not as big of a deal. My thinking started to change. I didn't have as many cravings during the week, but when I did, I only needed to remind myself, "This is a weekday; I don't have soda on weekday." Because I did not give myself a choice and didn't dwell on the fact that I couldn't have soda, the cravings lost their power over my thoughts.

When the third weekend came and went, on Monday I realized I hadn't had any soda on the weekend — I didn't even miss it. I gave myself few more weeks to fully adopt the rule of no soda Monday through 5 p.m. Friday before I started working on the next rule.

The next rule I worked on was to avoid any type of sweets or candy from Monday morning through 5 p.m. Friday. I set a clear definition of what I considered "sweets and candy," and got to work.

It has been over six years since I established these eating habits, and I now have a few sodas per month and some form of candy or sweets most weekends. The rule of "no sodas or candy during the week" is so ingrained in me that I hardly ever get any cravings during the week. My habit of not eating sweets on weekdays is so ingrained that if I'm at a birthday party during the week, I don't even feel the need to have cake (unless, of course, it's my own birthday). Ever since I made junk foods special, indulging in them on the weekends or special occasions only, I enjoy them much more. The best thing is, I don't feel guilty after I have them.

More importantly, I feel great during the week, which is when I have to be at my best. And, because I allow myself to indulge in some junk food every weekend, I don't feel deprived. Remember, your body can tolerate a certain amount of not-so-good food. As long as you eat healthfully the rest of the time and, of course, exercise regularly, you'll be able to maintain great health and a lean body. I am living proof of that.

The bottom line to my story is that learning to control *ourselves* is the only way we will be able to achieve our weight loss goals, because often our environment is not under our control.

In Section 8, I will show you, in 14 Simple Steps, how to make permanent changes in your eating habits, including how to make junk food special again. So who said you can't have your cake and eat it too?

# Section 6: More Weight Loss Mistakes

As I mentioned earlier, one of the biggest mistakes we make when trying to lose weight is trying to make too many changes in our lives at one time. Many weight loss programs tell us to make all those changes at once. In this section I will talk about two more common mistakes that sabotage countless weight loss efforts.

### Mistake #1: Loss of focus

Although most of us start a weight loss program with a goal in mind, as the program progresses we lose focus on our objective and the benefits we will reap by sticking to the program. Instead we start focusing on the discomfort of exercising, and feelings of deprivation such as missing our favorite TV shows because we have to go to the gym, or not being able to eat whatever we want.

As you know, we are a "NOW" society; we want everything *now*. We don't want to wait. So, the immediate pleasure of eating what we want *now,* or watching our favorite TV shows *now* usually wins over the benefits we will enjoy in the future if we go through some minor discomfort *now*. We are torn between the urge on the one hand, to indulge in minor pleasures *now* and avoid minor discomforts *now*, and, on the other hand, the goal of achieving major benefits in the future by going through those minor discomforts *now*. Unfortunately, in most cases, the first option wins.

### How to avoid making this mistake

You can avoid making the same mistake by creating a "trigger" to help you stay focused on your goal. What is a trigger? Have you ever heard a song that reminded you of a certain time in your life, or a certain place or person? The song is a "trigger" that brings back memories. Somehow, in your head, the song is linked with that certain place, person, or time in your life.

Here's how you can intentionally create a trigger to help you stay focused on your weight loss goal. Before you get started with any weight loss program, sit down in a quiet place and write down all the reasons why getting in shape and/or losing weight is important to you. How you are going to feel once you have achieved the body you want? How is getting fit going to affect your life and how other people see you? Keep writing all the benefits you hope to reap from getting in shape and/or losing weight. Don't be shy; write down as many as you can think of. No one but you needs to see this list.

Once you have completed the list, read it. As you do this, picture yourself already at your goal. How do you feel about yourself when you see yourself at the goal? How do other people feel about you? Maybe everybody who cares about you is proud — or even jealous! When you're at the peak of feeling great, do a small action, like pinching your thumb (or any other small action that can be easily done in public). Again, think about, and begin to feel, how great you'll look and feel when you have achieved your fitness goal, and pinch your thumb again. With your mind's eye, clearly see yourself at your fitness goal and keep pinching your thumb. Do this for at least for 10 minutes.

What you're trying to do is create a link between the everyday action of pinching your thumb and how you are going to feel when you have achieved your goal. It's the same concept as Ivan Pavlov's famous conditioning experiment. He got a dog to associate the ringing of a bell with the presence of food, so after a while the dog started salivating when it heard the bell, even when food was not present. We want to condition ourselves in the same way. Instead of the bell we'll use the pinching of our thumb (or whatever action you choose to use), and the automatic response we want is the feeling of well-being and accomplishment we'll feel when we achieve our fitness goals.

After you have created your trigger, practice it throughout the day. Keep practicing every day for one to two minutes, for at least 21 days straight. After that, the action of pinching your thumb will remind you of your fitness goals and how good you're going to feel when you have achieved them. As you start to apply the 8 Eating Rules into your life, you can use the trigger to help you get through cravings and stay focused on your fitness goals.

As a backup plan to help you stay focused, start another list of the negative effects you will experience if you continue with your current lifestyle habits. How are you going to look and feel one year from now if you continue the way you are, without making any lifestyle changes? How will your body look? How much might you weigh? How good or poor will your health be? How will other people see you? Picture yourself five years from now, 10 years from now, and 20 years from now — if you think you could live another 20 years with your current lifestyle. Don't leave any detail out. It may even help you to talk to people who didn't take care of their health when they were younger, and who now suffer because of it.

Take the two lists you created — the one you used to create your trigger, and the one that lists all the potentially negative effects of your current lifestyle — and put them aside. Look at both lists every weekend to remind yourself of the benefits you're working toward, and also the consequences of not sticking to your program.  During your weight loss program, when you find yourself focusing on the discomforts you're enduring in order to achieve your goals, pull out the two lists and read them. Remind yourself that you have a simple choice: you can endure minor discomforts now and reap the health benefits they'll lead to in the future, or you can continue as you are, and run the risk of suffering major discomforts from diseases (diabetes, heart disease, hypertension, etc.) that will most likely develop from an unhealthy lifestyle. It's your choice.  Knowing that may motivate you to stick to your weight loss program.

### Mistake #2:  Following an incomplete weight loss program

As you might already know, misinformation in the weight loss field sabotages countless efforts to lose weight and get in shape.  The biggest problem I find with most weight loss programs is that they offer only part of the solution to a weight problem.  No matter how well we follow an "incomplete" weight loss program, any results we get will not be permanent, or even sustainable.  For any weight loss program to be *complete*, it must include three things: some form of strength training, some form of aerobic activity, and it must not merely teach proper nutrition in terms of what to eat, but it should teach people how to make proper nutrition habitual.  Any weight loss program that does not include those three things is doomed to fail from the start.

How many times have you seen aerobic machines like steppers and treadmills promoted as though they are the only things needed for losing weight and getting a fit body?  If we were to follow that advice, we'd lose some weight initially. However, after a while the weight loss would stop.

Some aerobic equipment also offers a diet plan with it, so let's say we follow that diet and lose some more weight. Even then, the weight loss will stop after a while.

Why?  Because, when trying to lose weight by aerobics or aerobics and diet only, up to 25% of the weight that is lost is muscle.  As we lose muscle mass, our metabolic rate slows down, and we all know what happens when our metabolic rate slows down.  Weight loss stops unless we further reduce the calories that we take in.  By doing some form of resistance training as we are losing weight, we ensure that our body will maintain the muscle, which will keep our metabolic rate higher, which is good for losing weight. This is only one example of what happens when a weight loss program does not incorporate strength training, aerobic activity, and proper nutrition.

### How to avoid making this mistake

Make sure your weight loss program includes some form of strength training (free weights, Pilates, weight training machines, power yoga, etc.), some form of aerobics (treadmill, stepper, bike, walking outside, etc.), and proper nutrition (which you will learn in this book). The last and most important thing your weight loss program must have is a plan of action as to how you are going to incorporate all of the above into your life, without getting overwhelmed.

This book is part of your plan of action! In Section 8, I'll show you how to incorporate proper nutrition into your life in 14 Simple Steps.  If you need help making exercise a habit in your life, I suggest you buy my book, *Cracking the Weight Loss Code*, which you can purchase on my website, www.liveyourwaythin.com.

## Section 7: The 8 Eating Rules

Nutrition can be a very confusing subject. Every week, some new diet comes on the market, telling people the "best" way to eat. Even I, during my first 10 years in the fitness field, was very confused trying to figure out the best way to eat, not just for weight loss, but also for optimum health. Finally, I decided to look at cultures in which people lived very long, healthy lives. That's when I started looking at "Blue Zones" (author Dan Buettner's name for geographic areas where people live long and healthy lives) and realized that the typical Greek island diet, on which I was raised, is considered one of the healthiest diets on earth. As a matter of fact, the Greek island of Ikaria is considered one of the "Blue Zones." The diet and lifestyle on Ikaria is very similar to the way I was brought up on my home island of Evia. According to Dan Buettner, author of *The Blue Zones*, Ikaria is home to the highest percentage of people who live past 90 years of age.

I do realize that each of us is not able to live the same lifestyle as people who live on Ikaria or in other Blue Zones, but we can incorporate a lot of their habits into our lives. In this section, I will cover the eating habits — the 8 Eating Rules — you will need to develop.

Although there is more to proper nutrition than the 8 Eating Rules, if you make the 8 Eating Rules part of your lifestyle, not only will you lose all the weight you want, you'll also be much better off, health-wise, than you were before. Now let's take a look at the 8 Eating Rules.

# The 8 Eating Rules

## *Eating Rule #1: Don't eat unless you are physically hungry.*

This rule means that you shouldn't eat just to satisfy a craving. It also means you should not engage in preventive eating, which is the habit of eating when you have time to — even if you're not hungry — because you don't think you'll have time to eat later. One of the unhealthiest things we can do, which contributes the most to weight gain, is eating when we're not physically hungry. When you're not physically hungry, it means your body doesn't need any fuel at that time. If you eat when you're not hungry, most of the calories you consume at that time will be stored as fat. If you repeatedly find yourself in a situation where you have time to eat, but you're not hungry — but you eat anyway because you know you'll be hungry when you have no time to eat, keep fruit or nuts with you. Snack on them when you get hungry — not before!

Also remember, when you get hungry, you don't have to eat right away — unless, of course, you are diabetic. When you do get hungry, I suggest you have a glass of water and wait a little bit more before you eat. Being hungry is actually good for the body; it gives it a chance to use up some stored fat. Cravings, though hard to deal with, are not hunger. When you are truly physically hungry, you should have an "empty" feeling in your stomach, and maybe even hear some growling.

Here are more ways to tell the difference between physical hunger and cravings:

**You are most likely experiencing physical hunger when:**
a. All food tastes good, including your least favorite foods.
b. You have no doubt that you're hungry. (If you're "not sure" whether you're hungry, then you're not.)
c. You may feel "empty."
d. You may feel lightheaded.
e. You may feel weak.
f. You may feel a loss of energy.
g. You may feel a certainty that you must eat *now*.
h. All you want to do is eat. (If you feel like doing something other than eating, then you are not physically hungry.)

**You are most likely experiencing a craving when:**
a. You weren't hungry until you saw or smelled food.
b. You're searching your kitchen to find a food to satisfy a craving.
c. You just want to suck on or chew something.
d. You're feeling bored, angry, or anxious and you feel like eating something.
e. You're thirsty.
f. Your energy is low due to lack of sleep.

**Hunger is not an emergency**

Many of us are afraid to feel hunger. You can begin to lose this fear if you think of being hungry as a sign that your body is using its stored fat. If you keep supplying your body with fuel nonstop, by eating all the time, why would your body use up its stored fuel (body fat)? Our bodies always prefer to use up fuel that just came in (the food we eat), rather than breaking down and using its stored fuel (body fat). We must give our bodies a chance to use up stored fuel if we want to lose weight. Following Eating Rule #1 will help you do that. Get into the habit of asking yourself this question before you eat: "Do I want to eat because I am physically hungry, or is it for some other reason?" If the answer to this question is, "I am physically hungry," then go ahead and eat. If not, find something else do to.

*Eating Rule #2: Eat slowly and mindfully.*

This rule alone can help you lose weight. Studies have shown that people who eat more slowly eat less than people who eat faster. There are a couple of reasons why most people eat less when they eat slowly. One reason is, by eating more slowly, you give your brain a chance to register that you are full. It takes up to 20 minutes for your brain to get the message that your stomach is full. Additionally, by eating slowly and more mindfully, you'll feel more satisfied by the end of the meal, so you'll be less likely to ask for seconds.

Let me tell you a story my client Jim told me, which perfectly illustrates my point. Jim and his family had gone out to a restaurant to eat. That particular day, everybody was really hungry. Although the food was great, the service wasn't. First came the appetizers. After Jim and his family had finished their appetizers, the server took 20 minutes to bring their salads. After they had finished their salads, the server didn't bring their entrées for another 20 to 30 minutes.

Although everybody was very hungry when they first got to the restaurant, by the time the entrées came, everybody was full from having eaten only an appetizer and a salad. Usually, Jim said, he and his family could eat the appetizer, the salad, and the entrée with no problem. By simply waiting a little longer (even though it wasn't by choice), they felt full after having eaten less food. So you see, simply by eating more slowly, your brain has the chance to get the message that you are satisfied, allowing you to eat less and lose weight.

**Suggestions for eating more slowly and mindfully:**
1. Put down your fork between bites.
2. Be mindful of chewing your food. You can even count the number of bites silently, in your head. I suggest chewing each bite at least 10 times.
3. If you're eating a sandwich, always put down the sandwich between bites.

4. Never do anything else while eating (watching TV, having a meeting, playing games, having a serious conversation, etc.).
5. Drink some water every few bites.


### *Eating Rule #3: Eat the "right" amount of food.*

For many of us, eating "enough" food means feeling stuffed to the point where we can hardly move. For others of us, it means we must eat all the food on our plate, no matter how our stomachs feel. Others of us feel we must unbuckle our belts at least one notch. There are many definitions we use to denote the "right" amount of food. If you want to lose weight, you have to make sure you have a realistic definition.

My definition of the "right" amount of food is when I have eaten enough to satisfy my hunger, but I feel I could eat a little bit more. Keep in mind; it can take up to 20 minutes for your brain to get the message that you have eaten enough. That's why you should eat slowly and stop at a point where you feel you could eat a little bit more. Your stomach should not feel "stretched," and you should be able to take a brisk walk. If your stomach feels uncomfortable, you ate too much.

It worth noting that the citizens of Okinawa, Japan practice something called *hara hachi bu*, which means they eat until they feel only 80% full. According to Dr. Bradley J. Willcox, Dr. Craig Willcox, and Dr. Makoto Sukuzi, authors of *The Okinawa Diet,* the island of Okinawa has the highest occurrence of centenarians and the longest life expectancies in the world. In addition, Okinawans have one of the lowest rates of disease, from cancer to cardiovascular disease.

One of the reasons for the Okinawans' long, healthy lives, besides their consumption of mostly fruits vegetables and fruits and their low consumption of meats, is the low-calorie diet they eat. Eating slowly is one way that anybody can begin to "cut calories." Because Okinawans stop eating when they feel 80% full, they eat fewer calories per day for their body weight than we do here in the States. It's believed that eating less causes your body to builds fewer free radicals (unstable molecules that damage vital body molecules such as tissues, DNA, etc., and cause disease). Free radicals are generated mainly through the metabolizing of food into energy, so the less you eat, the fewer free radicals you build up.


### *Eating Rule #4: Make junk food special.*

Have junk food on weekends and special occasions *only*. Junk food is here to stay, but with this rule, you can learn to live with it and still lose weight. Don't worry about how you'll be able to eliminate junk food from your weekdays. There's a very simple way to achieve this, which I will describe in the next section.

*Eating Rule #5: Eat at least 4 servings of vegetables each day.*

Vegetables are excellent sources of vitamins, antioxidants, phytochemicals, minerals, and fiber. There is abundant evidence to support the notion that high intake of vegetables and fruits greatly reduces the risk of developing cancer, cardiovascular disease, inflammatory diseases, and many other chronic diseases. A diet high in fruits and vegetables is a must if you want to greatly improve your chances of living a long and healthy life.

*Eating Rule #6: Eat at least 3 or more servings of fruit each day.*

Here are more reasons why I think we should be eating more vegetables and fruits. A review of 200 epidemiological studies found that people who consumed diets high in fruits and vegetables had a 50 percent lower cancer risk, compared to people who ate only a few fruits and vegetables. Evidence substantially proves that high intake of fruits and vegetables greatly reduces the risk of chronic diseases such as cardiovascular heart diseases, diabetes, and certain cancers.

*Eating Rule #7: Eat at least one serving of beans/legumes at least 5 days each week, every day if possible.*

Why eat beans/legumes? For one thing, beans have been shown to have a cholesterol-lowering effect. Beans have a low glycemic index and, because of that, they play a positive role in preventing diabetes and obesity. In addition, beans appear to protect against cancer due to the phytochemicals and antinutrients they contain. There are great-tasting bean recipes in the Members' Section of my website, www.liveyourwaythin.com. Membership is free.

*Eating Rule #8: Don't eat more than 5 servings of meat or poultry each week.*

Most people have a very hard time following this rule. Many of us believe it's essential to have some form of meat every day. This can't be further from the truth, but there was once a time when even I believed it. At one point I was certified to teach a diet similar to the Zone Diet. Over the years, and after countless hours of reading nutritional studies and reports, I changed my mind. The one study that convinced me to eat less meat was the China Project, a study jointly conducted by researchers from Oxford University, Cornell University, and academic institutions in China. The China Project showed that, as consumption of animal products increased, so did cancer and heart disease. Animal products are essential to the diet, but not in large quantities. For more information on the China Project, go to www.nutrition.cornell.edu/ChinaProject/.

**There's more...**

Of course there's more to a health-enhancing diet than the 8 Eating Rules, but I think these are the most important rules, which will have the biggest effect on your weight and health. I suggest that you start your weight loss program by incorporating the 8 Eating Rules into your life and, once they have become second nature, you can make even more improvements in your diet. There are plenty of ideas on my website, www.liveyourwaythin.com, or my Olympus fan page on Facebook.

The 8 Eating Rules will not do you any good unless they become a part of your life. You can't just follow them once in a while and expect to get results. You'll need to make the 8 Eating Rules habitual, so you'll follow them automatically, without having to think about them. In the next section, I will show you, through 14 Simple Steps, how to start eating according to the 8 Eating Rules every day of your life.

# Section 8: 14 Simple Steps to Better Eating Habits

As I have said, the biggest mistake you can make when trying to change your eating habits is to try to make many changes at once. Regardless of any results you achieve, you will get overwhelmed and quit. So please follow the 14 Simple Steps slowly, and at your own pace. Each of the 14 Simple Steps outlined in this section will help you forge new eating habits in a meaningful, lasting way. Each step is designed to build upon the previous one, so please don't skip any steps unless the step you're working on asks you to do something you already do. For example, if the goal of a particular step is to get you to eat at least three vegetables per day, and you already do that, just skip that step and move to the next one.

### Motivation tip: Change your success indicator
To stay motivated, especially in the beginning when the weight might not be coming off as fast as you would like it to, you can keep yourself from getting discouraged by changing your success indicator.

Let me explain what I mean by that. Most of us, when we're trying to lose weight, use the scale as our success indicator. In other words, we weigh ourselves every week to see if the scale shows a lower number (which makes us feel successful) or a higher number (which makes us feel defeated). We can avoid motivation-destroying negative feelings by focusing not on the weight, but on the actions we're supposed to take in our weight loss program.

Let's say you are working on Step One (following Eating Rule #1 on Monday, Wednesday, and Friday). Additionally, you have a goal of doing three aerobic workouts and two strength training workouts that week. If you did all that, you had a successful week, *even if the number on the scale did not change*.

Nothing good comes out of using your weight as your success indicator. One problem with using weight as your success indicator is that sometimes you can do everything right, eat the perfect diet, do all your exercises, and the scale still doesn't move. This can happen for a multitude of reasons — eating salty food or a large meal before a weigh-in; for women, accumulated water weight during a menstrual cycle; or any number of other reasons. That's why it's more realistic and encouraging to focus on the habits you must develop in order to lose the weight you want.

So, at each step, make your success indicator the actions that you're asked to take. If you succeed in completing those actions, you had a successful week. Don't worry about the weight. If you follow the simple directions at each step, it's only a matter of time before the weight starts coming off.

**Further help**
I have created easy-to-use booklets that help track your progress at adapting each of the 8 Eating Rules into your life. You can purchase them on my website, www.liveyourwaythin.com.

**A word about weekends**
It's very important that you give yourself a break from the 8 Eating Rules on weekends. Sometimes I see people get so excited about losing weight, they want to follow the 8 Eating Rules every day. However, I've found over the years that people who are too strict burn themselves out. You must have one or two days each week when you can completely relax. Over time, you'll find that you're eating better, even on the weekends. If it happens, that's fine, but let it happen naturally. And, knowing you're allowed to eat what you want on the weekends will make it much easier to control yourself during the week. It's a way to make weekends even more special!

**Getting started**
Before you start on Step 1, you must develop a trigger that will remind you why you want to lose weight and get in shape. Having a strong trigger will be a big help in fighting off cravings as you go through each step. See Section 6 for detailed instructions on developing a trigger. Don't start on Step 1 until you have established your trigger.

# The 14 Simple Steps

## STEP 1

**Objective:** Follow Eating Rule #1 *(Don't eat unless you are physically hungry)* on Monday, Wednesday, and Friday.

The first Eating Rule is the most important rule. Make sure you are clear about the difference between physical hunger and cravings. If not, reread the rule in Section 7.

From now on, every Monday, Wednesday, and Friday, you will not eat unless you are physically hungry. Don't give yourself a choice. This is simply the rule you will live by from now on. On these three days, before you eat anything you must ask yourself, "Am I hungry?" If the answer is "no," or "not really," or if you're not sure, then don't eat. Eat only if you're absolutely positive that you are physically hungry. You don't have to follow the rule on Tuesday and Thursday, but don't go out of your way to break it, either.

*Tips:* I realize this rule might be hard for some people to follow, especially those of us who are prone to cravings, or who turn to food for comfort after a long, stressful day. The secret of breaking those bad habits is to give yourself no choice. By giving yourself no choice, and then choosing something else to do, other than eating, you will train yourself to avoid eating to relieve stress.

Choosing an activity other than eating is very helpful, and you'll be amazed at the solutions you can come up with. Some of my clients surf the web, play games on their cell phones, read a book, take a walk, or call a friend instead of eating to satisfy a craving or to de-stress. If you come up with a unique way of replacing stress eating with a more constructive activity, please let me know. You can e-mail me at stavros@liveyourwaythin.com.

### When to move to the next step

Move to the next step only when you have completed at least one perfect week. In other words, a week during which you only ate because you were hungry on Monday, Wednesday, and Friday. Even if you have completed two perfect weeks, you don't have to move to the next step until you feel ready. Take as much time as you like at each step. In fact, you're better off taking extra time at each step to make sure you're very comfortable with the Eating Rule you're working on, rather than trying to move through the steps too quickly, before you've truly established good habits.

## STEP 2

**Objective:** Build on Step 1 by following Eating Rule #1 *(Don't eat unless* *you are physically hungry)* perfectly the remaining two days of the week, Tuesday and Thursday.  So from Monday through Friday, you won't eat unless you're physically hungry.

**When to move to the next step**
Move to the next step only when you have completed at least one perfect week — preferably two.  In other words, you should have completed a week, Monday through Friday, during which you only ate when you were definitely physically hungry. Remember, you don't have to move to the next step until you feel comfortable doing so.

## STEP 3
**Objective:** Follow Eating Rule #2 (*Eat slowly and mindfully*) Monday, Wednesday, and Friday.  If you're not sure if you ate slowly and mindfully, you probably didn't.

*Tip:*  Don't pre-cut your food.  Cut one piece at a time and put down your knife and fork between bites. If you're eating a sandwich, put it down between bites. Chew a bite of food at least 10 times before swallowing (this is also good for digestion).  Pay attention to the flavors and textures of the food you're eating.

**When to move to the next step**
Move to the next step only when you have completed at least one perfect week. In other words, a week during which you ate every meal or snack slowly and mindfully on Monday, Wednesday, and Friday. Feel free to repeat this step until it becomes a habit. There's no rush to move on to the next step.

## STEP 4
**Objective:**  Build on Step 3 by following Eating Rule #2 (*Eat slowly and mindfully*) perfectly the remaining two days of the week, Tuesday and Thursday.  So from now on, Monday through Friday, you'll eat every meal or snack slowly and mindfully.

**When to move to the next step**
Move to the next step only when you have completed at least one perfect week — preferably two.  In other words a week, Monday through Friday, during which you ate every meal or snack slowly and mindfully.  Remember, even if you have completed two perfect weeks, you don't have to move to the next step until you feel absolutely ready to do so.

## STEP 5

**Objective:** Follow Eating Rule #3 *(Eat the "right" amount of food)* Monday, Wednesday, and Friday. Reread this rule in Section 7 to know exactly what the "right" amount of food is, and how to know when you've had enough.

*Tip:* Remember, it takes about 20 minutes for your brain to get the message that you are full. Stop eating at a point at which you feel you could eat more.

I would like to tell you a story one of my friends told me. He worked at a restaurant, and one day he was so busy he didn't get a chance to eat until late afternoon. By that point he was really hungry, so he made himself a big bowl of pasta. He had only six bites before the phone rang. Although he was still hungry, he had to take the call. He stayed on the phone for 30 minutes and, when he went back to finish his meal, he realized he was no longer hungry. Usually he ate a whole bowl of pasta before he felt satisfied — and also stuffed — but on this particular day he had only six bites and felt he was satisfied, without that stuffed feeling. His story perfectly illustrates my point; if you eat slowly, and stop eating at a point at which you feel you could eat more, you'll find that you feel perfectly satisfied, even though you've eaten less food than you might have eaten if you'd eaten at a faster rate.

### When to move to the next step

Move to the next step only when you have completed at least one perfect week. In other words, a week during which you did not overeat at any meal on Monday, Wednesday, and Friday

## STEP 6

**Objective:** Build on Step 5 by following Eating Rule #3 *(Eat the "right" amount of food)* the remaining two days of the week, Tuesday and Thursday. So from now on, Monday through Friday, you'll eat only until you are satisfied, not stuffed.

### When to move to the next step

Move to the next step only when you have completed at least one perfect week — preferably two. In other words, a week during which you did not overeat at any meal, Monday through Friday. Remember, even if you completed two perfect weeks, you don't have to move to the next step until you feel absolutely ready to do so.

### Review

By this time, you should be eating only when you are physically hungry, eating every meal and snack slowly and mindfully, and you should be able to stop eating at a point where you still feel slightly hungry, but satisfied. You should be able to do all of these things perfectly, Monday through Friday of every week.

By this point, you should be losing weight. If you aren't, you may not be following the rules as well as you think you are. Even if you're losing weight at a very good rate (one to two lbs. per week), don't stop here. Take a one-to-two-week break before moving on, to continue practicing Steps 1 – 6 and make sure the first three eating rules are habitual. Then move on to the next step.

The following steps will help you implement the remaining Eating Rules, which have to do with *what* you eat. These rules might help you speed up your weight loss a little bit more, but the main reason you want to incorporate them into your life is because they will have a big impact on improving your health. Remember, although losing weight and having a nice-looking body are great, enjoying good health and lowering your chances of developing deadly diseases is even better.

## STEP 7

**Objective:** Begin incorporating Eating Rule #4 *(Make junk food special)* into your life by eating junk food only on Tuesday, Thursday, and weekends.

Although eventually I want you to make junk food *very* special and have it on weekends and special occasions only, you shouldn't cut it down too fast. It will be easier to resist junk food on day if you know you can have it the next day, guilt free. Because Friday nights are often considered part of the weekend, many people have a difficult time not having any junk food on Friday night. My rule is, it's OK to have one serving of junk food on after 5 p.m. on Friday, if you really feel you have to have it. If you feel you need more help dealing with the desire to eat junk food, I'm working on a book specifically about junk food, *Let's Make Junk Food Special Again*, which will be available in 2011.

### Wine and beer
On the days when you're not supposed to have junk food, it's OK to have one small glass of wine or one bottle of beer if you really want to. More than one wine or beer is considered junk food, so you will be breaking the rule.

*Tip:* Do not remove junk food from your home. As I said in Section 5, you want to learn to control yourself, not your environment. If you have a strong craving, just remind yourself that you have no choice, and that you can indulge in the junk food you're craving the next day, when you can have it without feeling guilty. This is the time to use your trigger to remind yourself of your goals of a thinner body and increased health. Remember, dwelling on a craving gives it power over you. If you give yourself no choice, the craving loses its power.

**When to move to the next step**
When you have gone at least two weeks in a row without eating junk food on Monday, Wednesday, and Friday, you are ready to move to the next step.


## STEP 8
**Objective:** Build on Step 7, and make junk food even *more* special by eating it only on the weekends.

From now on, you will have no junk food from Monday morning through 5 p.m. Friday. As I said before, one small glass or wine or beer during the week is OK, as is one serving of junk food after 5 p.m. on Friday. You can enjoy junk food guilt-free on the weekends. However, if a holiday or special occasion such as an anniversary or your own birthday falls on a weekday, it's OK to have some junk food. After all, we want to make junk food special so you should be able to have it on special days.

**When to move to the next step**
When you have completed at least two weeks in a row of not having any junk food Monday, morning through 5 p.m. Friday, you are ready to move to the next step. Remember, if you don't feel quite ready to move on, it's OK to stay at this step until you feel you have fully implemented this habit.


## STEP 9
**Objective:** Apply Eating Rule #5 *(Eat at least 4 servings of vegetables each day)* on Monday, Wednesday, and Friday every week. (A serving is the size of your fist.)

*Tip:* Make a habit of having a good-sized salad before you eat dinner. The best dressing is olive oil and vinegar, but if you're going to have a creamy dressing, keep it on the side and dip your bare fork in it before you take a bite of your salad. Having a salad first will do two things: It will ensure that you get at least two servings of vegetables, plus it will curb your appetite a little so you will not overeat during dinner. Make sure your dinner also includes at least one vegetable.

You can get your fourth daily vegetable by carrying baby carrots, celery, or some other kind of vegetable with you to snack on if you get hungry. The key to getting more vegetables into your diet is to make them more available. You will find some delicious veggie recipes in Section 11 of this book.

**When to move to the next step**
Move to the next step when you have completed at least one week of eating at

least 4 servings of vegetables on Monday, Wednesday, and Friday. Repeat this step until eating four servings of vegetables on Monday, Wednesday, and Friday becomes a habit.

## STEP 10
**Objective:**  Eat at least 4 servings of vegetables every day of the week, including weekends.

**When to move to the next step.**
Move to the next step when you have completed at least one week — preferably two — of eating at least 4 servings of vegetables every day of the week.

## STEP 11
**Objective:** Apply Eating Rule #6 *(Eat at least 3 or more servings of fruit each day)* by having at least 3 or more servings of fruit each day every day of the week, including weekends.  (A serving is the size of an apple.)

*Tip:*  Always make sure you have your favorite fruits available at work and at home.  If you like a fruit that needs peeling or cutting, such as watermelon, cantaloupe, honeydew, etc. I suggest peeling and cutting it the night before, and placing it in a container to take it with you to work.

**When to move to the next step**
Move to the next step when you have completed at least one week of eating at least 3 fruits every day, including weekends.

## STEP 12
**Objective:**  Apply Eating Rule #7 *(Eat at least one serving of beans/ legumes at least 5 days each week, every day if possible)*.  (A serving of beans is ½ cup.)

*Tips:*  Beans are one of the few foods whose nutritional value improves with the canning process, so canned beans are OK to use.  Just make sure you rinse them, and try to select beans with low sodium.  I have included a few easy-to-make bean recipes in Section 11 of this book.  For more recipes, go to the Members' Section of my website, www.liveyourwaythin.com.  Membership is free.

**When to move to the next step**
Move to the next step when you have completed at least two weeks of eating at least one serving of beans, 5 days per week.

## STEP 13

**Objective:** Apply Eating Rule #8 (*Don't eat more than 5 servings of meat or poultry each week)*. (A serving is the size and thickness of your palm.) If you already don't have more than one serving of meat per day, skip to the next step.

*Tip:* Many people complain that they don't feel satisfied unless they eat some kind of meat at every meal. I suggest replacing some of your meat dishes with beans or fish. Either one will satisfy you as well as meat. If you are having a vegetarian dish, put some olive oil on it. Oleic acid, a fatty acid found in olive oil and other unsaturated fats, satisfies hunger just like meat does.

**When to move to the next step**
Move to the next step when you have completed two weeks of having one serving, or no servings, of meat every day of the week. You aren't allowed to have two servings of meat one day because you had none on a previous day.

## STEP 14

**Objective:** To implement Rule #8 (*Don't eat more than 5 servings of meat or poultry each week)* perfectly. You can have all 5 servings of meat in two meals, or in five meals; it's your choice.

**Where to go from here**
If you stick with everything you learn in these 14 Simple Steps, you should be able to keep off all the weight you lose. If you have not yet achieved your weight loss goal, as long as you stick with the 8 Eating Rules — and, of course, keep exercising — you'll keep losing weight until your body gets to the weight it was meant to be. If you're interested in making further improvements in your diet, become a member of my website at www.liveyourwaythin.com and you'll receive updates on the latest developments in diet and exercise. Membership is free.

# Section 9: More Nutritional Advice

**Breakfast is NOT the most important meal of the day**

I don't think breakfast is the most important meal of the day. Here is my reasoning. First of all, when I lived in Greece, breakfast was a very small meal, if it was eaten at all. This is true in many European nations. My second problem with breakfast is that most people aren't even hungry in the morning, and we now know it's not a good idea to feed your body when it isn't hungry. There's a reason why most people are not hungry in the morning: The body is trying to detoxify itself.

According to Ori Hofmekler, author of *The Warrior Diet*, your body, through the food you eat and through the air you breathe, accumulates toxins which, if they accumulate in large enough amounts, will make you sick. Avoiding all toxins is impossible, so the next best thing you can do is give your body a chance to detoxify on a daily basis. We can do that by giving our bodies long periods without eating. If you eat during this process, detoxification stops, because now the body needs to shift gears to digest the food we just ate.

According to Harvey and Marilyn Diamond, authors of the bestseller *Fit For Life*, between the hours of 4 a.m. and noon, your body is going through a detoxification process, and eating a heavy breakfast will interfere with this process. Of course if you *are* hungry in the morning, and you have made sure the feeling you're experiencing is physical hunger and not cravings or habit, do eat, but keep your meal light; don't have bacon and eggs. If you must eat in the morning, keep it small: fruit, or a small bowl of oatmeal or yogurt.

**Eat lightly during the day**

I know this advice goes against what most nutritionists recommend, but let me explain why I think eating lightly is usually the best way for most of us to eat.

As I said, in Greece we used to have a very light breakfast (if we ate breakfast at all). Then we had a big lunch and a small dinner, which was more like a large snack. After the big lunch, however, we had three hours to relax or take a nap

45

— a luxury we don't have here in the States. It is very important that you get to relax after a big meal, to aid digestion.

Think about this. How do you feel after you eat a big meal? You *want* to relax or take a nap, right? In Greece, every fall we used to go to my grandfather's village to collect olives. We'd get up early in the morning, collect olives all day, and not get home until sunset. During that time, we ate a light lunch and had a big dinner. You see, although lunch was usually our biggest meal, when we had to work through the afternoon, lunch became a small meal and dinner became the largest one. I think we did that instinctively, knowing that if we ate a big lunch, we wouldn't have the energy to collect olives all afternoon.

In America today, we work through the day and we don't have the luxury of a three-hour lunch break. Since most of us only get to relax at the end of the day, that's when we should have our biggest meal.

If you get hungry during the day, I suggest eating a light lunch of mostly vegetables. If you like a dessert at lunchtime, have fruit. By keeping lunch light, and eating mostly vegetables and fruits, you won't tax your digestive system and you won't get the "low" that many people feel in the afternoon, after a big lunch. Other benefits of fruits and vegetables (especially raw ones) include the vital nutrients they provide, such as enzymes, vitamins, minerals, and phytochemicals that aid detoxification — and also the digestion of the heavier meal you'll have at the end of the day. For more information on the benefits of eating light during the day and having your largest meal at the end of the day, I recommend reading *The Warrior Diet* by Ori Hofmekler.

**About whole grains**
Whole grains do play an important role in health, but overeating them could contribute to obesity and weight gain. If you're going to have grain products like bread, bagels, cereals, etc., I recommend that you choose whole grain products. I don't have any specific recommendation on how many servings of whole grains one should have; one or two servings per day might not be a bad idea.

**About dairy products**
Dairy foods do have their benefits, especially fermented dairy foods such as yogurt, cottage cheese, and kefir. These fermented foods contain probiotics that are beneficial to our health. Though I don't think we need to drink milk as adults, I do recommend that people eat at least one serving of a fermented dairy product every day, or at least most days of the week. Although they are not well understood yet, probiotics play an important role in overall health, including the health of your gastrointestinal track and your immune system.

**How much water should we drink?**
I've heard different numbers as to how many glasses of water one should drink each day. In truth, the answer depends on what types of foods you consume. If your diet is made up of foods that have a high water content, like fruits and

vegetables, and you don't eat a high amount of salt, you may be able to drink only three or four glasses of water each day. But if you eat a typical American diet high in meats, salt, and highly processed foods and low in fruits and vegetables, you might need to drink eight to 10 glasses of water per day. Of course, if you're very active, especially aerobically, drink more water.

I recommend that you drink at least six to eight glasses of water per day, more if you are very active, especially in hot weather. When you've established all of the 8 Eating Rules, you're eating foods with a higher water content, and can cut your water consumption to around five to six glasses of water per day.

Although minimizing the use of salt is ideal, if you're eating a diet high in salt, I recommend that you drink at least eight to 10 glasses of water per day, more if you are active.

## About artificial sweeteners

I don't recommend artificial sweeteners. Studies like one done in 1997 by J.H. Lavin, S.J. French, and N.W. Read, at the Centre for Human Nutrition, Northern General Hospital, Sheffield, U.K. suggest that people who use artificial sweeteners like aspartame make up for the calories they didn't consume due to the artificial sweetener, by eating more calories later. I have not seen a study that showed substituting sugar with artificial sweeteners made any difference in people's weight. The best thing to do is do cut down the amount of sugary beverages or foods you eat overall. If you're going to have a sweet treat, make sure it contains real sugar, not a substitute. We don't yet know all the effects artificial sweeteners can have on the body.

## About coffee

If you're going to drink coffee, have it before noon and try not to have more than two cups per day. Drinking coffee later in the day will interfere with your sleep. Even if it doesn't keep you up at night, coffee does make you a light sleeper and it will affect the quality of sleep negatively. Not sleeping well or not sleeping enough has been shown to increase appetite the next day.

## About weight loss drugs

Remember, to lose weight permanently you need to make permanent changes in your diet and exercise habits. Even if you found a drug that could really help you lose weight, you'd need to stay on it forever if you wanted to keep the weight off forever. The minute you went off the drug, the weight would come back.

All the weight loss drugs I'm aware of have side effects and were not meant for long-term use. How many times have you heard of some miracle new weight loss drug, only to hear about the drug's terrible side effects a few months later? Remember, the root causes of your weight problem are your dietary and exercise habits. Weight loss drugs only mask those problems; they don't fix anything. If you want to fix your weight loss problem forever, you must change the habits that made you overweight in the first place.

### About dietary fats

Dietary fat isn't a problem if you follow the first three Eating Rules. As long as you've made it a habit to eat only when you're hungry, to eat slowly and mindfully, and eat just "enough" food, even if you eat something that contains a considerable amount of fat, you'll find that you satisfy your hunger sooner, and you won't eat as much. It will also take you longer to get hungry again.

I can give you a personal example. If I have a salad for lunch (no meat, just vegetables) tossed with a little bit of olive oil and vinegar, I get hungry again after four or five hours, but if I have a slice of pizza for lunch I can go for at least seven hours before I get hungry again. The extra fat in the pizza satisfies my hunger for a much longer period.

The only fats I recommend avoiding are trans fats. Saturated fats, although you do want to limit them, are not as bad as trans fats. Besides, you'll cut down on your consumption of saturated fats naturally once you apply Eating Rule #8 (Don't eat more than 5 servings of meat or poultry each week) into your life.

Olive oil and flaxseed oil are the best fats. When making a salad or cooking a vegetarian meal, don't be afraid to use olive oil. Most of the Greek vegetarian dishes I was raised on had plenty of olive oil in them. Just make sure you eat only when you are hungry, eat slowly and mindfully, and stop eating when you have satisfied your hunger.

# Section 10: A Few Words on Exercise

Although this book is about how to improve your diet so you can lose weight and improve your health, I want to make sure you realize that exercise plays a very important role in weight loss and health as well. The two forms of exercise you should include in your weight loss program are some form of strength training and some form of aerobic activity.

### Why strength train?
Did you know that the average adult over the age of 25 loses four pounds of muscle every 10 years? That happens because the body does not like waste. At all times, it tries to conserve energy and get rid of anything it doesn't need, like extra muscle that it doesn't use. Since most people don't use their muscles for strenuous work on a regular basis, the body gets rid of the muscle it doesn't need.

Also, muscles themselves conserve energy by only utilizing the smallest number of fibers needed to complete a task. Let me explain. A muscle, depending on its size, is made up of hundreds of thousands of muscle fibers. The fibers are the units that contract and produce the power. If you don't need a lot of power, your muscle will recruit only a small number of fibers, in order to conserve energy. Have you seen that new eight-cylinder Buick, which can drive on only four cylinders when you don't need the extra power? Your muscles do pretty much the same thing.

Let me give you an idea about how muscle can affect your weight. Your body is burning calories at all times, even when you are not doing anything. This is your resting metabolic rate. Some people have a higher resting metabolic rate, which means they are burning more calories, even at rest. Some people have a lower resting metabolic rate, which means they are burning fewer calories at rest. One of the factors that determines your resting metabolic rate is the amount of muscle you have. In other words, the more muscle you have, the more calories you burn. Depending on which study you read, one pound of muscle burns anywhere from 20 to 30 calories a day in its resting state.

Let's say you started strength training and gained four pounds of muscle. This means you will burn an extra 80 to 120 calories per day, and that's in a resting state. You can lose an extra eight to 12 pounds of fat in a year simply by gaining four pounds of muscle. If you become active by doing aerobics, having more muscle means you will burn more calories.

Now, the problem with losing muscle as we age is the fact that it affects our metabolic rate, and as our metabolic rate gets slower and slower, we gain weight unless we change our eating habits. Most people notice weight gain around the age of 30, because by that time they have lost enough muscle to slow down their metabolic rate to the point where they begin gaining weight.

Since our everyday lives don't require much heavy lifting, we need to give our bodies a reason to maintain existing muscle, or to add more muscle. That is where strength training comes in. It provides the stimulus the body needs to maintain and/or build muscles. Maintaining muscle mass is essential for maintaining a higher metabolic rate, which makes weight loss easier.

Here is one more fact that you'll find very interesting, if you want to lose weight. Studies have shown that when people lose weight by dieting and aerobic training only, up to 25% of the weight they lose comes from muscle, which in turn slows down your metabolic rate and makes weight loss more difficult. Basically, trying to lose weight without doing some form of resistance training is a great way to sabotage your progress. Even if you don't gain any muscle from strength training, your metabolic rate will still increase, due to the fact that you'll stimulate your muscles to recruit more muscle fibers, which will make you stronger and, more importantly, the muscle itself will utilize more calories, which will help you lose weight.

**Need help with starting a strength training workout?**
You can find more information on strength training and how to start a strength training workout in the Members' Section of my website, www.liveyourwaythin. com. Membership is free.


**The importance of aerobic training**
Aerobic exercise is any exercise that requires oxygen for the production of energy. The reason aerobic exercise is important to a weight loss program is that it's one of the fastest ways to burn fat, and the fastest way to improve your cardiovascular system, which is very important to overall health and well-being. Moreover, by improving your cardiovascular system, you become more aerobically fit and your body is better able to burn stored fat.

Keep in mind that even though aerobics offers great benefits, doing aerobics without doing anything else can actually sabotage your progress. For example, you can be doing plenty of aerobics and still gain weight because you're not watching your diet. Or, as I mentioned earlier, if you're trying to lose weight by doing aerobics only, up to 25% of the weight you will lose will come from muscle.

Try to stretch after each workout, to prevent your muscles from stiffening up. Hold each stretch for 15 seconds or more. The following are examples of indoor and outdoor aerobic exercises. *Outdoors:* Walking, jogging, cycling, cross-country skiing, hiking, swimming, inline skating, rowing. *Indoors:* Treadmill, stair-stepper, stationary cycle, NordicTrack, rowing machine, swimming, aerobics classes.

If you're wondering which aerobic workout burns the most calories, it doesn't really matter. All that matters is that you choose an aerobic activity you like, because the bottom line is, if you don't like a particular aerobic activity, you won't do it consistently, even if it's the "best" exercise you can do. Nor will you push yourself while you're doing it, so you won't get the maximum benefit from it anyway. So when it comes to picking aerobic activities, don't try to choose the one that burns the most calories, choose the one you enjoy the most.

I advise my clients to start with three aerobic workouts per week of 10 to 20 minutes each and work their way up to three to five aerobic workouts per week of 30 minutes each.

I'm in the process of writing a new book that covers everything you need to know about exercise and how to make exercise habitual, in the same way this book will help you make good eating habits second nature. If you'd like updates on my new book, become a fan of Olympus Personal Training & Weight Management on Facebook.

# Section 11: Healthy Recipes

I encourage you to experiment with these recipes; try different vegetables, quantities, and spices to match your taste. The vegetable quantities are all estimates. Have fun making these recipes your own!

### *Cannellini Bean Salad*

1 lb. cannellini beans, fresh or canned (if fresh, soak in water overnight, then boil until soft)

5 scallions, chopped

3 red and/or green peppers, chopped

2 oz. olive oil (or to taste)

vinegar (to taste, optional)

pinch salt


Mix vegetables and beans, add olive oil and vinegar to taste.

Use as much or as little of each ingredient as you like, according to your taste. Don't use too much olive oil because, although a little is good for you, too much is still fattening. This salad will stay fresh very well in the refrigerator and you can eat it cold. Make it in large amounts and have it throughout the week.

## *Broccoli & Red Pepper Soup*

2 lbs. fresh or frozen broccoli, chopped into large pieces

2 sticks celery, coarsely chopped

1 large onion, diced

3 garlic cloves, finely chopped

3 Tbsp. dried vegetable soup mix (such as Vogue VegeBase)

1/3 cup uncooked brown rice

3 red bell peppers

juice from 1 lemon

1 Tbsp. vinegar

seasonings (to taste, but very little salt)

### Step 1

In a large soup pot, combine 3 quarts of water, broccoli, celery, onion, garlic, vegetable soup mix, and rice. Simmer, covered, until broccoli is soft.

### Step 2

Cut the red peppers in half and remove the seeds. Roast under a broiler or on a grill, skin side facing the heat source, until skin begins to blacken. Remove the skins and puree peppers in a blender.

### Step 3

When the broccoli is soft, mash the vegetables in the pot using a potato masher. Add pureed red peppers to the pot. Add lemon, vinegar, and seasonings (e.g., tarragon, thyme, white or black pepper) to taste.

## Artichoke Hearts with Peas

3 lbs. canned artichoke hearts, cut in half

4 cups frozen peas, thawed

handful fresh dill, chopped

6 scallions, chopped

1 ½ cups tomato sauce (fresh or canned)

2 Tbsp. olive oil

1 cup water (more as needed)

salt (to taste)

pepper (to taste)

### Step 1

Sauté dill and scallions in olive oil for 5 minutes.

### Step 2

Add the peas, and sauté for 5 more minutes.

### Step 3

Add the tomato sauce, artichoke hearts, water, pepper, and very little salt. Cook until artichokes are hot.

-

### Black-Eyed Pea Salad

*For this salad, select quantities of the vegetables according to your taste.*

black-eyed peas (fresh or canned; if fresh, soak in water overnight, then boil until soft)

onions, chopped

scallions, chopped

tomatoes, chopped

romaine lettuce, finely chopped

fresh dill, chopped

olive oil (to taste)

vinegar (to taste, optional)

pinch salt

Mix all vegetables with peas. Add olive oil and vinegar to taste.

Use as much or as little of each ingredient as you like. Just make sure you don't use too much olive oil because, although it is good for you, too much is still fattening. This salad will stay fresh in the refrigerator and can be eaten cold. You can make it in large amounts and have it throughout the week.

-

### *Boiled Chicory Salad*

*This great side dish is easy to make and is very good for you. It can be eaten hot or cold, so you can make it ahead of time and keep it in the refrigerator.*

1 bunch chicory

olive oil (to taste)

lemon juice (to taste)

pinch salt

**Step 1**

Cut the root off the chicory and wash the chicory.

**Step 2**

Boil in slightly salted water until the stem is soft (about 30 minutes).

**Step 3**

Strain chicory, cut into bite-sized pieces.

**Step 4**

Add olive oil, lemon juice, salt. Mix and serve.

-

### Mediterranean-Style Lima Beans

1 lb. bag dry lima beans (soak in water overnight)

2 cups tomato sauce

2 Tbsp. olive oil

1 medium onion, chopped

2 cloves garlic, chopped

3 Tbsp. fresh parsley, chopped

oregano (to taste)

pinch salt

pepper (to taste)

**Step 1**

Boil beans with a little salt, until they are soft, but not too soft (about 45 minutes).

**Step 2**

Heat oven to 350 degrees. Put olive oil in a skillet and sauté the onions, garlic, and oregano 3 to 4 minutes. Add the parsley, salt, pepper, and tomato sauce, and continue cooking another 10 minutes.

**Step 3**

Once beans are done, drain them, *reserving some of the cooking liquid.*

**Step 4**

Put the beans in an ovenproof pan and add the tomato mixture.

**Step 5**

Add reserved water from the boiled beans, until beans are nearly covered. Mix and put in the oven for about 40 minutes.

-

## *Peas & Corn*

1 onion, chopped

2 cloves garlic, chopped

3 cups mushrooms, any variety, diced

1 can peeled whole tomatoes in juice, chopped

2 cups frozen peas, thawed

1 cup frozen corn, thawed

oregano (to taste)

1 Tbsp. olive oil

black pepper (to taste)

pinch salt

bay leaves (1 if whole, a pinch if chopped)

### Step 1

Put olive oil in large pan and sauté the onions and garlic for 3 minutes.

### Step 2

Add mushrooms and sauté for 3 minutes.

### Step 3

Add chopped tomatoes with the juice. Add oregano, black pepper, salt, and bay leaves. Bring to a boil.

### Step 4

Once boiling, add peas and corn and cook 10 to 15 minutes, uncovered, until peas and corn are cooked.

## *Ratatouille*

1 eggplant, cubed

2 zucchini, cubed

2 green and/or red peppers, diced large

1 large onion, diced

1 medium-sized can whole tomatoes, coarsely chopped

2 Tbsp. olive oil

1 clove garlic, chopped

oregano (to taste)

pepper (to taste)

pinch salt

### Step 1

Sauté onions with the olive oil, garlic, salt, pepper, and oregano, until onions are translucent.

### Step 2

Add the tomatoes and cook 5 minutes.

### Step 3

Add the eggplant and cook for about 10 minutes.

### Step 4

Add the zucchini and peppers and cook until the vegetables are done.

-

## Red Beet Salad

This easy-to-make side dish is very good for you.  It can be eaten hot or cold, so you can make it ahead of time and keep it in the refrigerator.

1 bunch fresh beets with their greens

olive oil (to taste)

vinegar (to taste)

pinch salt

### Step 1

Peel the beets and cut them in halves or quarters, depending on how big they are.

### Step 2

Wash beet greens, put them in a pot with the beets, and fill with water.

### Step 3

Boil until beets are fork-tender (about 30 minutes). Strain and put beets and greens in a bowl.

### Step 4

Add little olive oil, vinegar to taste, a little salt, and mix._

### Spinach & Rice

4 lbs. spinach, stems removed

handful fresh dill, chopped

9 scallions, chopped

4 Tbsp. olive oil

7 cups tomato juice

2 cups chicken stock

1 14-oz. box instant brown rice

oregano (to taste)

pinch salt

pepper (to taste)

**Step 1**

In a large pot, sauté the scallions and dill in the olive oil.

**Step 2**

Add the oregano, salt, pepper, brown rice. Sauté 1 minute.

**Step 3**

Add the tomato juice and chicken stock, bring to a boil, and stir in the spinach. Reduce heat and simmer covered, stirring occasionally to prevent sticking (*Note: if you are using thawed frozen spinach, wait until the rice is almost cooked before adding it.*) Cook until the rice is done.

-

## *Spinach with Onions*

1 lb. spinach

1 large onion, thinly sliced

2 cloves garlic, finely chopped

1 Tbsp. olive oil

oregano (to taste)

pepper (to taste)

pinch salt

### Step 1

In a pot, sauté the onions and garlic in the olive oil until onions are translucent.

### Step 2

Add the spinach and the spices, and cook until spinach is done.

-

### Greek-Style Tomato Salad

2 ripe tomatoes, cut in wedges

1 green pepper, thinly sliced

½ red onion, thinly sliced

oregano (to taste)

salt (to taste)

3 Tbsp. olive oil (or to taste)

2 slices feta cheese (optional)


Mix ingredients in a bowl and serve.  If possible, allow the salad to sit for 30 minutes to allow the flavors to mingle.

-

## *Eggplant & Beans (main course)*

1 eggplant, peeled and diced

1 onion, thinly sliced

1 green pepper, diced

1 Tbsp. lemon juice

3 Tbsp. ketchup

very little olive oil

2 cups garbanzo or other beans, cooked or canned

½ onion, finely chopped (optional)

**Step 1**

Steam the eggplant for 10-12 minutes. (If you don't have a steamer, put eggplant in a pot with a little water and cover. Make sure you stir it often so it won't stick.)

**Step 2**

Wet a napkin with a little olive oil and wipe the cooking surface of a pan with it. Sauté the sliced onion and pepper over low heat in a covered skillet for 6-8 minutes.

**Step 3**

Add the steamed eggplant, lemon juice, and ketchup and simmer, uncovered, another 5 minutes. Add the beans, cook until hot, and add the chopped onion right before you take the skillet off the heat.

-

### Mushroom & Onion Mix (side dish)

3 cups mushrooms, any variety, diced

1 onion, diced

1 to 2 Tbsp. dried vegetable soup mix such as Vogue VegeBase (to taste)

Wet a napkin with a little olive oil and wipe the cooking surface of a pan with it. Sauté the onions and mushrooms 5 minutes and add the vegetable soup mix. Cook until done.

### Eggplant Patties (main course or side dish)

2 eggplants, peeled and sliced

3 Tbsp. balsamic vinegar

4 cloves garlic, finely chopped

1 cup fat-free, low sodium vegetable stock

1 Tbsp. rosemary, finely chopped

pinch black pepper

pinch oregano

1 Tbsp. Bragg's Liquid Aminos

**Step 1**

Heat oven to 350 degrees. Slice eggplant into 1/3 inch thick patties.

**Step 2**

Mix the remaining ingredients in a flat-bottomed bowl.

**Step 3**

Wet a napkin with a little olive oil and wipe down a nonstick baking tray or sheet of aluminum foil, creating a thin coating of oil.

**Step 4**

Dip the eggplant patties in the spice mixture for 5 seconds, then place on the oiled tray or foil.

**Step 5**

Bake eggplant for 20-25 minutes. Mushrooms can be used instead of, or in addition to, the eggplant.

### Dip for Eggplant Patties (optional)

½ cup fat-free or 50% reduced fat mayonnaise

Garlic, finely chopped (to taste)


Mix the mayonnaise and garlic.


*Tip:* Do not dip the vegetables directly into the dip because you'll end up with too much. Instead, dip the tip of your bare fork in the dip, and eat your vegetables with it. This way, you'll get the taste of the dip, without overpowering the vegetables or consuming too much fat.

-

### Vegetable Scrambled Eggs

2 eggs (free range or organic)

8 oz. Rancho Fiesta Style Vegetables, thawed

1 cup feta cheese, cut in small cubes

½ cup onions, chopped

½ cup tomatoes, chopped

1 Tbsp. olive oil

salt (to taste)

pepper (to taste)

**Step 1**

Heat olive oil in a pan and add the chopped onions.  Cook 4 minutes.

**Step 2**

Add the chopped tomatoes.  Cook 2 minutes.

**Step 3**

Add the thawed vegetables and cook until hot. (Cover the pan to heat the vegetables faster.)

**Step 4**

Beat the eggs in a bowl, mix in the feta cheese, and add mixture to pan.  Season with salt and pepper.  Keep mixing until eggs are fully cooked.

*Note:* To reduce the fat, remove one of the egg yolks before you beat the eggs.

### Spinach Salad with Tuna

4 ½ oz. fresh baby spinach

1 cup water-packed canned tuna

1 cup diced cucumber

½ cup canned corn

¼ cup chopped scallions

1 Tbsp. olive oil

1 Tbsp. balsamic vinegar


Mix ingredients in a large bowl and serve.

### Village-Style Black-Eyed Pea Salad

2 cups canned black-eyed peas, rinsed and well drained (if using fresh beans, soak in water overnight, then boil until soft)

2 cups diced red pepper

1 cup diced cucumber

½ cup chopped scallions

¼ cup chopped dill

2 Tbsp. olive oil

2 Tbsp. vinegar

salt (to taste)

Mix ingredients in a large bowl and serve.

-

### Romaine Lettuce Salad with Dill

1 head romaine lettuce

1 cup chopped scallions

½ cup chopped fresh dill

2 Tbsp. olive oil

2 to 3 Tbsp. vinegar (to taste)

salt (to taste)

**Step 1**

Cut romaine lettuce thinly, on the diagonal.

**Step 2**

Mix ingredients in a large bowl and serve.

# Section 12: Conclusion and Final Thoughts

There are no secrets to losing weight and getting in shape. There is no magic pill that will help you lose weight, nor will there ever be one. The truth is, weight loss will take some effort on your part. Only permanent changes in your daily habits will result in permanent weight loss. In order to lose weight and get into shape, all you need to do is implement a balanced resistance training routine (two to three times per week), an aerobic training routine (four to five times per week), and the 8 Eating Rules I introduced in this book. You have to be consistent in your efforts if you want to get results.

Any weight loss program that does not include strength training, aerobic training, and proper nutrition is doomed to fail. A program that promises weight loss with little or no effort on your part is deceiving you. If it were that easy to lose weight, everybody would be thin by now. Keep in mind that weight loss is not everything. Being healthy is far more important. Losing weight in an unhealthy way will only harm you in the long run.

Confucius said, "A journey of a thousand miles begins with a single step." A journey of a thousand miles can seem overwhelming, but when you focus on one single step at a time, it becomes a much easier proposition. Your journey toward achieving a lean and healthy body begins with changing a single habit.

Let me tell you a story that perfectly demonstrates how focusing on one small step can make a big difference in your life. As you might already know, many people have a hard time flossing regularly. Despite the fact that flossing is very beneficial and doesn't take more than five minutes, most people don't seem to be able to stick to the task regularly. For years, I was one of these people. I would go to my dentist for a cleaning and he'd lecture me on the importance of flossing and all the bad things that could happen to my teeth if I didn't floss regularly. I'd leave the dentist's office determined to start flossing every night from then on.

But once I got home, I'd floss regularly for few weeks and then, for whatever reason, I'd stop. At my next checkup, it would be the same routine. The dentist would tell me that if I didn't floss enough, bad things would happen to my teeth, I'd get motivated for few weeks, but then I would stop flossing again. This went on for years.

One day I thought to myself, how am I supposed to motivate people to develop good exercise and eating habits, when I can't even get myself to stick to the habit of flossing daily? The answer came to me when I came across the kaizen method, which helps people implement change in their lives through small, easy steps.

Kaizen is a Japanese word that means, "change for the better." The kaizen method was first used in Japan after World War II, by companies like Toyota, in an attempt to improve all functions of the company by taking small but continuous steps. We all know how well Japanese industry — especially the automobile industry — did after World War II. The kaizen method played a big part in that rapid turnaround. I decided I would try the kaizen way to get myself flossing regularly.

I started flossing one tooth every night. I must admit, I did feel a little silly flossing only one tooth, but I stuck to my task. Night after night, I flossed one tooth. Every person I told about my strange new habit told me that I wasn't getting any benefit from flossing only one tooth. My response was that I was not trying to floss, I was trying to *develop the habit* of flossing, and by keeping the action so small, it was almost impossible not to do it. Every so often, when I felt like it, I'd add one more tooth to floss. One day I realized I was flossing every tooth! It's been five years since then, and flossing has become an automatic action that I do every night without a second thought.

If you want to lose weight and keep it off permanently, good eating habits also have to become automatic. The only way to make good eating habits automatic is to introduce them into your life one at a time, just like I did with flossing one tooth at a time. Once you've made good eating habits automatic, you'll never have to worry about your weight again, thanks to your new way of healthful eating.

If you have any questions or comments about my program, please don't hesitate to e-mail me at stavros@liveyourwaythin.com. I look forward to hearing your success story!

# For Further Reference and Reading

American Council on Exercise. *Personal Trainer Manual.* San Diego, CA: American Council on Exercise, 1996.

Ballentine, Rudolph. *Diet and Nutrition: A Holistic Approach.* Honesdale, PA: The Himalayan Institute Press, 1978.

Beck, Judith S. *The Beck Diet Solution*, 2007. Birmingham, AL: Oxmoor House, 2007.

Cordain, Loren. *The Paleo Diet.* New York: John Wiley and Sons, 2002.

Diamond, Harvey. *The Fit for Life Solution.* St Paul, MN: Dragon Door Publications, 2002.

Diamond, Harvey and Marilyn. *Fit For Life.* New York: Warner Books, 1985.

Faigin, Rob. *Natural Hormone Enhancement.* Cedar Mountain, NC: Extique Publishing, 2000.

Fuhrman, Joel. *Eat To Live.* New York: Little, Brown and Company, 2003.

Hofmekler, Ori. *The Warrior Diet.* St Paul, MN: Dragon Door Publications, 2001.

Maltz, Maxwell. *The New Psycho-Cybernetics.* New York: Prentice-Hall, 2001.

Maurer, Robert. *One Small Step Can Change Your Life: The Kaizen Way.* New York: Workman, 2004.

Roizen, Michael. and La Puma, John. *The Real Age Diet.* New York: HarperCollins, 2001.

Tilden, J.H. *Toxemia Explained.* Pomeroy WA: Health Research Books, 1960.

# Acknowledgments

First, I would like to thank the most important people in my life: My wife Svetlana, my son Alexander, and my daughter Arina, for their understanding and support while I was writing this book. I worked many long days trying to finish it, which took away a lot of our time together.

Another person to whom I owe everything to is my mother, Iris Mastrogiannis, who supported me through all the ups and downs of my life and my career. I would also like to thank the rest of my family, the Rountos and Beretis, because without their support my personal training business might not even exist.

Many people have helped in the creation of my weight loss program and in the writing of *The 8 Eating Rules*. I would especially like to thank my clients at Olympus Personal Training & Weight Management, because without their input and the trust they put in me, this book would never have been written. The other person I would like to thank is Becky Schoenfeld for the great job she did editing this book and for going beyond what I expected from her. She was a great influence on the look and feel of this book.

The following people, although I have never met them in person, have had a great impact on my life. Their inspiration, through their books and tapes, has kept my motivation alive throughout the seemingly endless research that went into developing and writing *The 8 Eating Rules*. Thank you, Anthony Robbins and Robert Allen.

*About the Author*

**Stavros Mastrogiannis**

**Founder & Personal Trainer, Olympus Personal Training & Weight Management**

Stavros Mastrogiannis, founder of Olympus Personal Training & Weight Management Center in Danbury, Connecticut, is a 17-year veteran in the weight loss field, empowering clients with a unique, life-changing perspective. Stavros resided in Greece for 12 years before moving to the United States in 1987. After moving to the U.S., Stavros continued to visit Greece where, over time, he observed changes in Greek eating habits, exercise habits, and daily living, resulting in a national weight problem similar to that which exists in the U.S.

At age 21, Stavros made the decision to shift gears, from the pursuit of a career in felt he could make a difference in peoples' lives. He is committed to preparing fine cuisine, to the weight loss and fitness profession, where he putting an end to widespread weight loss misinformation, and to helping people lose weight the healthy way.

Stavros founded Olympus Personal Training & Weight Management Center in 1996. His approach to fitness stresses the importance of developing a realistic regimen of exercise and nutrition that can be maintained for a lifetime of good health. His exceptional understanding of motivation and consistency as the root of success in long-term fitness has enabled him to teach hundreds of people how to effectively lose weight and keep it off, even when other trainers and diet plans have failed.

Stavros provides his clients with cutting-edge nutrition and weight loss information from the top medical institutes. He is a source of inspiration for thousands, having organized the Danbury Weight Loss Challenge in 2004 and having partnered with St. Jude Children's Hospital in Memphis, TN for the Get In Shape for 2007 Challenge.

Prior to founding Olympus Personal Training & Weight Management Center, Stavros was a fitness instructor for the Regional YMCA of Western Connecticut and Newtown Health & Fitness Club. In these positions, Stavros enjoyed educating, training, and motivating his clients as they pursued their weight loss and fitness goals.

Stavros holds an A.O.S. in Culinary Arts from the Culinary Institute of America. He received a diploma in Fitness and Nutrition from International Correspondence Schools and holds numerous certifications, including CPR, Nutrition Specialist, and ACE (American Council on Exercise) certifications as a Personal Trainer and Lifestyle & Weight Management Consultant.